LOW-FODMAP COOKBOOK FOR SENIORS(40+)

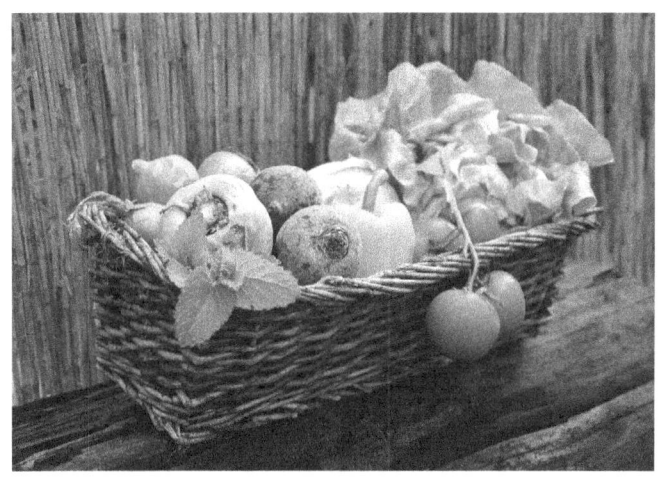

Delicious and Digestion-Friendly Recipes for Happy Seniors

CHRIS WILLIAM

COPYRIGHT

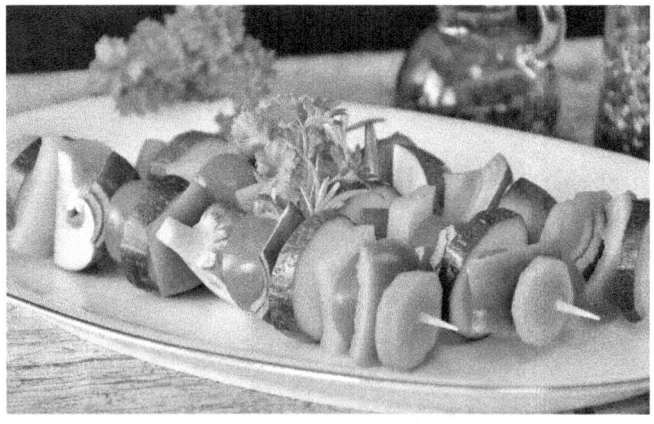

TABLE OF CONTENT

INTRODUCTION

Mrs. Thompson had always enjoyed cooking for her family and friends, but in recent years, she had started to experience uncomfortable symptoms whenever she ate certain foods. She often felt bloated, had stomach cramps, and felt fatigued. It was becoming more and more challenging for her to prepare meals that didn't trigger these unpleasant reactions.

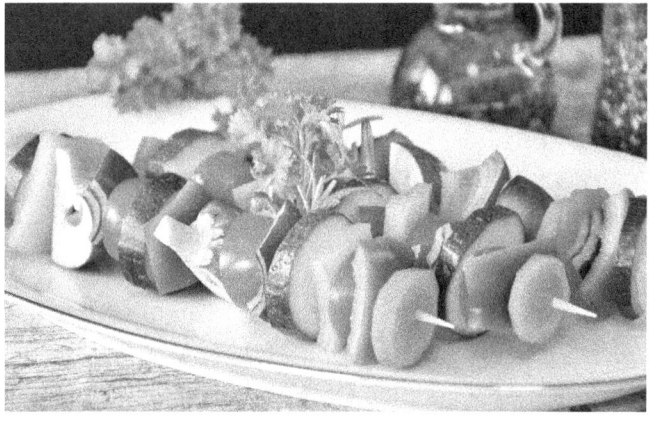

One day, while at her doctor's appointment, Mrs. Thompson learned about the low FODMAP diet. The doctor explained that it was a way of eating that could help reduce the symptoms of irritable bowel syndrome (IBS), which Mrs. Thompson had been experiencing. Essentially, it involved avoiding certain types of foods that can be difficult for some people to digest, such as lactose, fructose, and certain types of carbohydrates.

Mrs. Thompson was eager to try the low FODMAP diet, but she was worried about how she would manage to cook meals that were both healthy and delicious. She was also concerned about how she would find the energy and motivation to experiment with new recipes.

That's when she discovered the Low FODMAP Cookbook for Seniors. This book was specifically designed to help seniors like her eat well and reduce the symptoms of IBS. The book was filled with easy-to-follow recipes that were low in FODMAPs, yet still flavorful and satisfying. It also included tips on meal planning, grocery shopping, and how to adapt favorite recipes to fit within the low FODMAP guidelines.

With the help of the cookbook, Mrs. Thompson was able to enjoy cooking and eating again, without worrying about the unpleasant symptoms that had been plaguing her. She felt more energetic, healthier, and happier knowing that she was taking care of her body in a way that was both practical and delicious.

WHAT ARE FODMAP

FODMAPs (Fermentable Oligosaccharides, Disaccharides, Monosaccharides, and Polyols) are a group of short-chain carbohydrates and sugar alcohols that are commonly found in many different types of foods. These compounds are not well absorbed in the small intestine, which can lead to digestive symptoms in some people, particularly those with irritable bowel syndrome (IBS) and other functional gastrointestinal disorders.

FODMAPs can be found in many different types of foods, including wheat, dairy products, fruits, vegetables, legumes, sweeteners, and some processed foods. Some of the most common sources of FODMAPs include wheat, onions, garlic, beans, lentils, cabbage, broccoli, cauliflower, apples, pears, peaches, watermelon, honey, and high fructose corn syrup.

When consumed, FODMAPs can pass through the small intestine without being fully absorbed. As they reach the large intestine, these carbohydrates can be fermented by bacteria, which produces gas and other byproducts. This fermentation process can lead to a range of digestive symptoms, including bloating, abdominal pain, diarrhea, and constipation.

To help alleviate these symptoms, a low FODMAP diet may be recommended for individuals with IBS and other digestive disorders. This diet involves limiting the intake of high-FODMAP foods, while still maintaining a balanced and nutritious diet.

WHAT IS A LOW FODMAP DIET

A low FODMAP diet is a type of dietary approach that is designed to help manage symptoms of irritable bowel syndrome (IBS) and other functional gastrointestinal disorders. The term "FODMAP" stands for Fermentable Oligosaccharides, Disaccharides, Monosaccharides, and Polyols, which are a group of short-chain carbohydrates and sugar alcohols that can be difficult for some people to digest.

The low FODMAP diet involves temporarily restricting the intake of high FODMAP foods, while still maintaining a balanced and nutritious diet. This is typically done in three phases:

1. Elimination phase: During this phase, high FODMAP foods are eliminated from the diet for 2-6 weeks. This helps to reduce symptoms and allows the gut to heal.

2. Reintroduction phase: After the elimination phase, individual FODMAPs are gradually reintroduced into the diet, one at a time, to

identify which specific types of FODMAPs may be triggering symptoms.

3. Personalization phase: Once trigger foods have been identified, the individual can then personalize their diet to include a balance of low FODMAP foods, as well as those that are well tolerated.

The goal of the low FODMAP diet is to identify and eliminate foods that are high in FODMAPs and causing symptoms, while still maintaining a healthy and balanced diet. The diet is not intended to be a long-term solution, but rather a temporary approach to help manage symptoms while other treatment options are explored.

Foods that are typically restricted on a low FODMAP diet include:

- Wheat, rye, and barley
- Dairy products containing lactose
- Certain fruits, such as apples, pears, peaches, and watermelons
- Certain vegetables, such as onions, garlic, broccoli, cauliflower, and cabbage
- Legumes, such as beans and lentils
- Sweeteners, such as honey and agave syrup

- Some processed foods that contain high fructose corn syrup or other high FODMAP ingredients

Foods that are typically allowed on a low FODMAP diet include:

- Gluten-free grains, such as rice, quinoa, and oats
- Lactose-free dairy products, such as lactose-free milk and hard cheeses
- Low-FODMAP fruits, such as bananas, blueberries, and strawberries
- Low-FODMAP vegetables, such as carrots, green beans, and bell peppers
- Protein sources, such as meat, fish, and eggs
- Nuts and seeds
- Certain herbs and spices

WHO SHOULD FOLLOW A LOW-FODMAP

If you're someone who experiences symptoms of irritable bowel syndrome (IBS) or other functional gastrointestinal disorders, you may have heard about the low FODMAP diet. This dietary approach has gained popularity in recent years as a way to manage symptoms such as bloating, abdominal pain, diarrhea, and constipation. But who exactly should follow a low FODMAP diet, and is it the right approach for you?

The low FODMAP diet is typically recommended for individuals who have been diagnosed with IBS or other functional gastrointestinal disorders. These conditions can cause a wide range of symptoms that can be difficult to manage, and the low FODMAP diet has been shown to be an effective way to reduce symptoms and improve quality of life for many individuals.

In addition to IBS, the low FODMAP diet may also be recommended for individuals with other digestive disorders, such as inflammatory bowel disease (IBD), small intestinal bacterial overgrowth (SIBO), and gastroesophageal reflux disease (GERD). It may also be beneficial for those with non-gastrointestinal conditions such as fibromyalgia and chronic fatigue syndrome.

However, it's important to note that not everyone with digestive issues will benefit from a low FODMAP diet. In fact, for some individuals, following a low FODMAP diet may not be necessary or even appropriate. For example, if you have been diagnosed with a food allergy or intolerance, it's important to address that specific issue rather than following a more general dietary approach like the low FODMAP diet.

If you're considering following a low FODMAP diet, it's important to work with a trained healthcare professional, such as a registered dietitian. A healthcare professional can help you to determine if a low FODMAP diet is appropriate for your individual needs and to ensure that you are following the diet safely and effectively. They can also help you to identify any underlying causes of your digestive symptoms and develop a comprehensive treatment plan that is tailored to your individual needs.

In conclusion, the low FODMAP diet can be a valuable tool for managing symptoms of IBS and other functional gastrointestinal disorders. However, it's important to work with a healthcare professional to determine if the diet is appropriate for you and to ensure that you are following the diet safely and effectively. If you're experiencing digestive symptoms, it's important to seek medical advice in order to identify any underlying conditions and develop an appropriate treatment plan.

BENEFITS

The low FODMAP diet has been shown to provide several benefits for individuals who experience symptoms of irritable bowel syndrome (IBS) and other functional gastrointestinal disorders. Some of the potential benefits of a low FODMAP diet include:

1. **Reduced symptoms:** One of the main benefits of a low FODMAP diet is a reduction in symptoms such as bloating, abdominal pain, diarrhea, and constipation. This is because FODMAPs can be difficult to digest for some individuals, leading to fermentation in the gut and the production of gas and other byproducts that can cause symptoms.

2. **Improved quality of life:** By reducing symptoms, the low FODMAP diet can also improve an individual's overall quality of life. This can include improvements in social, emotional, and physical well-being.

3. **Personalized approach:** The low FODMAP diet is a personalized approach that can be tailored to an individual's specific needs and preferences. This can

help to ensure that the diet is sustainable and effective in managing symptoms.

4. **Identification of trigger foods:** Following a low FODMAP diet can also help to identify trigger foods that may be causing symptoms. Once these trigger foods are identified, they can be reintroduced into the diet in a controlled manner to determine which foods are problematic and which can be consumed without issue.

5. **Reduced reliance on medications:** For some individuals, following a low FODMAP diet can reduce their reliance on medications to manage symptoms. This can be especially beneficial for those who experience side effects from medications or who prefer to manage symptoms through dietary changes.

It's important to note that the low FODMAP diet is not intended to be a long-term solution. Once symptoms have been managed and trigger foods have been identified, a healthcare professional can work with an individual to develop a more balanced and varied diet that meets their nutritional needs and preferences.

Overall, the low FODMAP diet can provide significant benefits for individuals with IBS and other functional gastrointestinal disorders. However, it's important to work with a trained healthcare professional to ensure that the diet is safe and effective for your individual needs, and to ensure that your nutritional needs are being met.

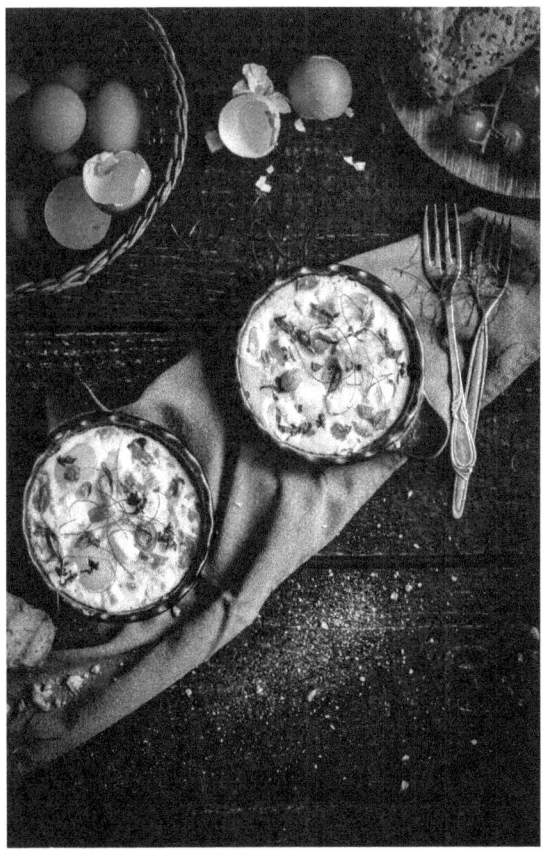

BREAKFAST

Gluten-Free Oatmeal with Blueberries and Almonds:

Ingredients:
- 1/2 cup gluten-free rolled oats
- 1 cup water
- 1/2 cup blueberries
- 1 tbsp chopped almonds

Steps:
1. In a small saucepan, bring the water to a boil.
2. Add the rolled oats and reduce heat to medium-low.
3. Stir occasionally for about 5-7 minutes, until the oats are cooked and the mixture has thickened.
4. Remove from heat and transfer to a bowl.
5. Top with blueberries and chopped almonds.

Low FODMAP Smoothie Bowl:

Ingredients:
- 1 medium ripe banana, peeled and frozen
- 1/2 cup frozen strawberries
- 1/2 cup unsweetened almond milk
- 1 tbsp chia seeds

- 1 tbsp unsweetened coconut flakes

Steps:
1. In a blender, combine the frozen banana, frozen strawberries, and almond milk.
2. Blend on high speed until smooth.
3. Pour the smoothie into a bowl.
4. Top with chia seeds and coconut flakes.

Scrambled Eggs with Spinach and Tomatoes:

Ingredients:
- 2 large eggs
- 1 cup baby spinach
- 1/2 cup cherry tomatoes, halved
- 1 tbsp olive oil
- Salt and pepper to taste

Steps:
1. In a small bowl, whisk together the eggs with salt and pepper.
2. Heat the olive oil in a non-stick skillet over medium heat.
3. Add the spinach and cherry tomatoes to the skillet and cook for 2-3 minutes, until the spinach is wilted and the tomatoes are slightly softened.

4. Pour the eggs into the skillet and scramble until cooked.
5. Serve immediately.

Gluten-Free Banana Pancakes:

Ingredients:
- 1 ripe banana, mashed
- 2 eggs
- 1/4 cup gluten-free flour
- 1/4 tsp baking powder
- 1/4 tsp vanilla extract
- 1 tbsp maple syrup (optional)

Steps:
1. In a mixing bowl, combine the mashed banana, eggs, gluten-free flour, baking powder, and vanilla extract.
2. Mix well until the batter is smooth.
3. Heat a non-stick skillet over medium heat.
4. Spoon about 2-3 tablespoons of batter onto the skillet for each pancake.
5. Cook for 2-3 minutes on each side, until golden brown.
6. Drizzle with maple syrup, if desired.

Low FODMAP Greek Yogurt Parfait:

Ingredients:
- 1/2 cup lactose-free Greek yogurt
- 1/4 cup fresh raspberries
- 1/4 cup gluten-free granola
- 1 tbsp chopped walnuts

Steps:
1. In a small bowl, layer the Greek yogurt, raspberries, and granola.
2. Top with chopped walnuts

Quinoa Breakfast Bowl with Berries and Nuts

Ingredients:
- 1 cup cooked quinoa
- 1/4 cup mixed nuts (e.g. almonds, pecans, walnuts), chopped
- 1/4 cup fresh berries (e.g. strawberries, raspberries, blueberries)
- 1 tbsp honey (optional)

Steps:
- In a small bowl, mix together the cooked quinoa and chopped nuts.
- Top with fresh berries and drizzle with honey, if desired.

Low FODMAP Smoothie:

Ingredients:
- 1 medium ripe banana, peeled
- 1/2 cup frozen blueberries
- 1/2 cup unsweetened almond milk
- 1 tbsp almond butter
- 1 tsp chia seeds

Steps:
1. In a blender, combine the banana, frozen blueberries, almond milk, almond butter, and chia seeds.
2. Blend on high speed until smooth.
3. Pour into a glass and serve immediately.

Turkey Sausage Breakfast Sandwich:

Ingredients:
- 1 gluten-free English muffin, toasted
- 1 cooked turkey sausage patty
- 1 large egg
- 1 slice of lactose-free cheddar cheese
- Salt and pepper to taste

Steps
1. Heat a non-stick skillet over medium heat

2. Crack the egg into the skillet and sprinkle with salt and pepper
3. Cook the egg until the white is set, but the yolk is still runny
4. Meanwhile, heat the turkey sausage patty according to package instructions
5. Assemble the sandwich by placing the cooked egg, turkey sausage patty, and cheese on one half of the toasted English muffin
6. Top with the other half of the English muffin and serve immediately.

Low FODMAP Breakfast Burrito

Ingredients
- 1 gluten-free tortilla
- 2 large eggs, scrambled
- 1/4 cup diced bell peppers
- 1/4 cup shredded cheddar cheese
- 1 tbsp salsa (check label for low FODMAP ingredients)
- Salt and pepper to taste

Steps:
1. Heat a non-stick skillet over medium heat.
2. Add the diced bell peppers and cook until slightly softened, about 2-3 minutes.

3. Add the scrambled eggs to the skillet and cook until fully cooked.
4. Place the tortilla on a plate and top with the scrambled eggs, bell peppers, cheddar cheese, and salsa.
5. Fold in the sides of the tortilla and roll up to form a burrito.
6. Serve immediately.

Low FODMAP Banana Bread:

Ingredients
- 1 1/2 cups gluten-free flour
- 1/2 tsp baking powder
- 1/2 tsp baking soda
- 1/2 tsp ground cinnamon
- 1/4 tsp salt
- 3 ripe bananas, mashed
- 1/2 cup lactose-free milk
- 1/4 cup maple syrup
- 1/4 cup melted coconut oil
- 1 large egg

Steps:
1. Preheat the oven to 350°F.
2. In a mixing bowl, combine the gluten-free flour, baking powder, baking soda, cinnamon, and salt

3. In a separate mixing bowl, combine the mashed bananas, lactose-free milk, maple syrup, melted coconut oil, and egg.
4. Mix well until the mixture is smooth.
5. Add the dry ingredients to the wet ingredients and mix until well combined.
6. Pour the batter into a greased loaf pan.
7. Bake for 45-50 minutes, or until a toothpick inserted into the center of the bread comes out clean.
8. Allow the bread to cool in the pan for 10 minutes before transferring to a wire rack to cool completely.

Low FODMAP Omelette:

Ingredients:
- 2 large eggs
- 1/4 cup diced bell peppers
- 1/4 cup diced tomatoes
- 1/4 cup shredded lactose-free cheddar cheese
- Salt and pepper to taste
- 1 tbsp chopped fresh chives (optional)

Steps:
1. Heat a non-stick skillet over medium heat.
2. Whisk the eggs together in a small bowl and season with salt and pepper.

3. Add the diced bell peppers and tomatoes to the skillet and cook until slightly softened, about 2-3 minutes.
4. Pour the eggs into the skillet and cook until the bottom is set, about 2-3 minutes.
5. Sprinkle the shredded cheddar cheese over the top of the omelette and fold the omelette in half.
6. Cook for an additional minute or until the cheese is melted.
7. Top with chopped fresh chives, if desired.

Low FODMAP Breakfast Hash:

Ingredients:
- 1 medium sweet potato, peeled and diced
- 1/2 cup diced bell peppers
- 1/2 cup diced zucchini
- 2 cooked turkey sausage links, sliced
- 1 tbsp olive oil
- Salt and pepper to taste

Steps:
1. Heat a large skillet over medium heat.
2. Add the olive oil to the skillet and heat until hot.
3. Add the sweet potato to the skillet and cook until slightly softened, about 5-7 minutes.

4. Add the diced bell peppers and zucchini to the skillet and cook until all the vegetables are tender, about 5-7 minutes.
5. Add the sliced turkey sausage to the skillet and cook until heated through.
6. Season with salt and pepper to taste.
7. Serve hot.

Low FODMAP Peanut Butter and Jelly Toast:

Ingredients:
- 2 slices gluten-free bread, toasted
- 2 tbsp peanut butter
- 2 tbsp low FODMAP jelly (e.g. strawberry, raspberry, grape)

Steps:
1. Spread peanut butter on one slice of the toasted bread.
2. Spread low FODMAP jelly on the other slice of the toasted bread.

3. Sandwich the two slices of bread together.
4. Serve immediately.

Low FODMAP Green Smoothie:

Ingredients:
- 1 medium ripe banana, peeled
- 1/2 cup frozen pineapple chunks
- 1/2 cup fresh spinach
- 1/2 cup unsweetened coconut milk
- 1 tbsp shredded coconut

Steps:
1. In a blender, combine the banana, frozen pineapple chunks, fresh spinach, coconut milk, and shredded coconut.
2. Blend on high speed until smooth.
3. Pour into a glass and serve immediately.

Low FODMAP Yogurt Parfait:

Ingredients:
- 1/2 cup lactose-free plain Greek yogurt
- 1/4 cup low FODMAP granola
- 1/4 cup fresh strawberries, sliced
- 1 tbsp maple syrup

Steps:
1. In a bowl or jar, layer the Greek yogurt, low FODMAP granola, and sliced strawberries.
2. Drizzle with maple syrup.

3. Serve immediately.

Low FODMAP Banana Pancakes:

Ingredients:
- 1 ripe banana, mashed
- 2 large eggs
- 1/4 cup gluten-free oat flour
- 1/4 tsp baking powder
- 1/4 tsp vanilla extract
- Pinch of salt
- 1 tbsp coconut oil

Steps:
1. In a medium bowl, whisk together the mashed banana and eggs.
2. Add the oat flour, baking powder, vanilla extract, and salt to the bowl and stir until well combined.
3. Heat a non-stick skillet over medium heat.
4. Add the coconut oil to the skillet and heat until hot.
5. Spoon 1/4 cup of the pancake batter onto the skillet for each pancake.
6. Cook until bubbles form on the surface of the pancakes, about 2-3 minutes.
7. Flip the pancakes and cook until lightly browned on the other side, about 1-2 minutes.

8. Serve hot with your favorite low FODMAP toppings, such as maple syrup or fresh fruit.

Low FODMAP Breakfast Burrito:

Ingredients:
- 1 gluten-free tortilla
- 2 large eggs
- 1/4 cup diced bell peppers
- 1/4 cup diced tomatoes
- 2 slices cooked bacon, chopped
- 1 tbsp chopped fresh cilantro
- Salt and pepper to taste

Steps:
1. Heat a non-stick skillet over medium heat.
2. Whisk the eggs in a small bowl and season with salt and pepper.
3. Add the diced bell peppers and tomatoes to the skillet and cook until slightly softened about 2-3 minutes.
4. Add the chopped bacon to the skillet and cook until heated.
5. Pour the eggs into the skillet and cook until scrambled about 2-3 minutes.
6. Warm the gluten-free tortilla in the microwave for 10-15 seconds.

7. Spoon the scrambled eggs onto the center of the tortilla.
8. Top with chopped fresh cilantro.
9. Roll up the tortilla and serve immediately.

Low FODMAP Shakshuka:

Ingredients:
- 2 large eggs
- 1/4 cup diced bell peppers
- 1/4 cup diced tomatoes
- 1/4 tsp ground cumin
- 1/4 tsp paprika
- Pinch of cayenne pepper
- Salt and pepper to taste
- 1 tbsp chopped fresh parsley (optional)

Steps:
1. Heat a non-stick skillet over medium heat.
2. Add the diced bell peppers and tomatoes to the skillet and cook until slightly softened, about 2-3 minutes.
3. Stir in the ground cumin, paprika, and cayenne pepper and cook for an additional minute.
4. Crack the eggs into the skillet, spacing them apart.
5. Season the eggs with salt and pepper.

6. Cover the skillet and cook until the eggs are set, about 3-5 minutes.
7. Sprinkle with chopped fresh parsley, if desired.
8. Serve hot with gluten-free bread or pita.

FISH AND SEAFOOD

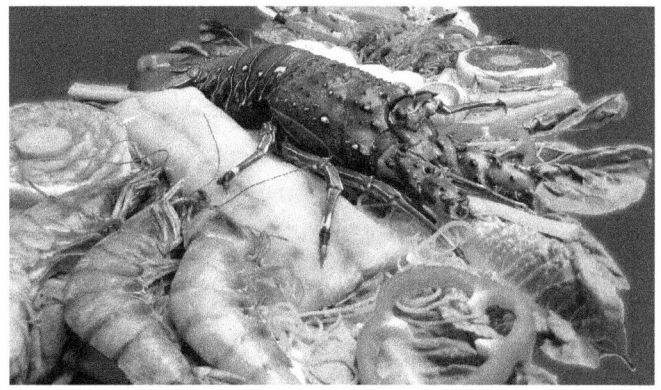

- Anchovies
- Cod
- Crab
- Haddock
- Halibut
- Lobster
- Mackerel
- Mahi-mahi

- Salmon
- Sardines
- Scallops
- Shrimp
- Sole
- Tilapia
- Trout
- Tuna

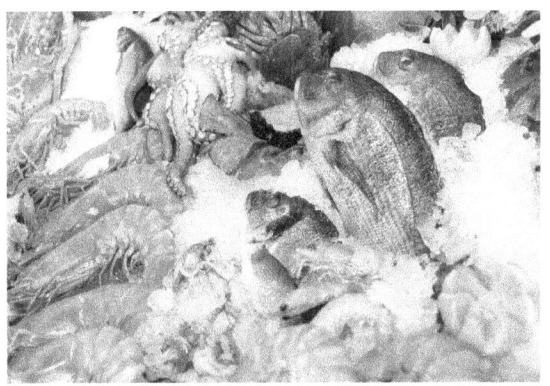

It's important to note that serving sizes can affect the FODMAP content of a food, so be sure to check appropriate serving sizes for each food. Additionally, some forms of seafood (such as canned or processed) may contain added ingredients that are high in FODMAPs, so it's important to read labels carefully.

VEGETARIAN AND VEGAN

Here are some low FODMAP vegetarian and vegan options:

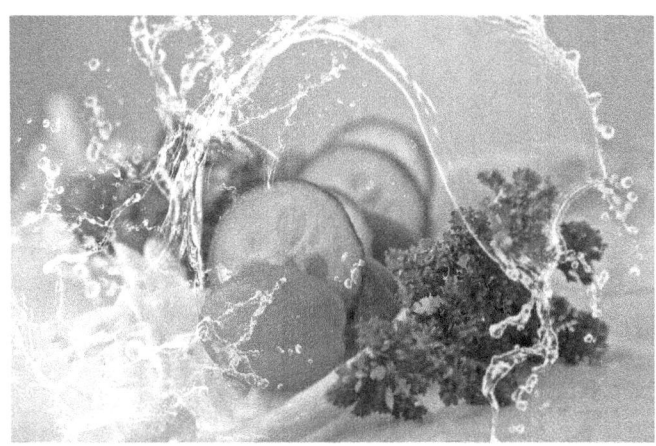

Protein sources:

- Tempeh (up to 1/2 cup)
- Tofu (up to 1/2 cup)
- Quinoa (up to 1 cup cooked)
- Brown rice (up to 1 cup cooked)
- Canned lentils (up to 1/2 cup)
- Canned chickpeas (up to 1/4 cup)
- Canned black beans (up to 1/4 cup)
- Firm polenta (up to 1/2 cup)
- Nuts and seeds (up to 1/4 cup)

Vegetables:

- Bell peppers (up to 1 cup)
- Carrots (up to 1 medium)
- Cucumbers (up to 1/2 cup)

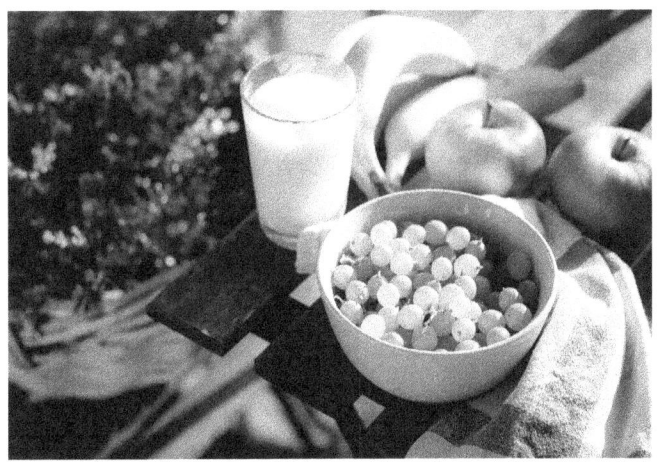

- Green beans (up to 1 cup)
- Lettuce (up to 2 cups)
- Olives (up to 15 small)
- Tomatoes (up to 1 cup)

Fruits:

- Bananas (1 medium)
- Blueberries (up to 1/4 cup)
- Grapes (up to 1 cup)
- Kiwi (1 medium)
- Oranges (1 medium)
- Pineapple (up to 1/2 cup)

- Raspberries (up to 1/4 cup)
- Strawberries (up to 1/2 cup)

Fats:

- Olive oil (up to 1 tablespoon)
- Coconut oil (up to 1 tablespoon)
- Flaxseed oil (up to 1 tablespoon)
- Macadamia nut oil (up to 1 tablespoon)
- Walnuts (up to 1/4 cup)

It's important to note that serving sizes can affect the FODMAP content of a food, so be sure to check appropriate serving sizes for each food.
Additionally, some vegetarian and vegan products (such as faux meat, seitan, or soy-based products) may contain high FODMAP ingredients, so it's important to read labels carefully.

SNACKS AND DESSERTS

Snacks:

- Rice cakes with peanut butter or almond butter
- Gluten-free pretzels
- Carrot sticks or cucumber slices with hummus
- Popcorn (plain or lightly salted)

- Roasted almonds or other low FODMAP nuts
- Hard-boiled eggs
- Cheese sticks or slices (cheddar, swiss, etc.)
- Low FODMAP protein bars or shakes (check labels for ingredients)
- Turkey or chicken slices with low FODMAP veggies (e.g. cherry tomatoes, bell peppers)

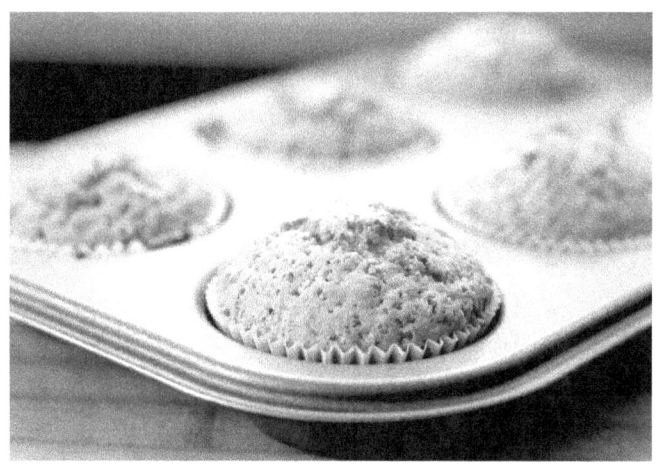

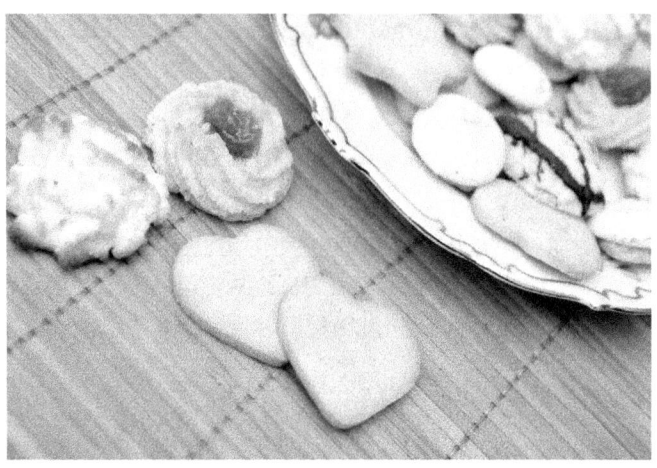

Desserts:

- Dark chocolate (check for no high FODMAP ingredients)
- Low FODMAP fruit with lactose-free yogurt or whipped cream (e.g. strawberries, raspberries, blueberries, kiwi)
- Gluten-free oatmeal cookies (made with low FODMAP ingredients)
- Rice pudding (made with lactose-free milk)
- Peanut butter or almond butter cups (made with dark chocolate and low FODMAP sweeteners)
- Low FODMAP cheesecake (made with lactose-free cream cheese and low FODMAP sweeteners)
- Banana bread (made with gluten-free flour and low FODMAP sweeteners)

- Lemon bars (made with gluten-free flour and low FODMAP sweeteners)

As always, it's important to check the labels and ingredients of any pre-made snacks or desserts to ensure they are low FODMAP. Additionally, portion control is important when it comes to snacks and desserts, so be mindful of how much you're consuming.

MEAT RECIPES

Grilled Chicken with Lemon and Thyme: Marinate boneless chicken breasts in olive oil, lemon juice, fresh thyme, salt, and pepper for a few hours. Grill the chicken until fully cooked, and serve with a side of grilled vegetables.

Steak Fajitas: Marinate thinly sliced sirloin steak in lime juice, cumin, smoked paprika, salt, and pepper for at least an hour. Saute the steak with bell peppers and onions, and serve with corn tortillas.

Beef and Broccoli Stir-Fry: Cook sliced beef in a wok or skillet with garlic-infused oil. Add broccoli florets, sliced carrots, and a low FODMAP stir-fry sauce (e.g., soy sauce, rice vinegar, and maple syrup). Serve over rice or quinoa.

Baked Turkey Meatballs: Mix ground turkey with breadcrumbs, egg, parsley, salt, and pepper. Form into balls and bake in the oven until fully cooked. Serve with a low FODMAP marinara sauce and zucchini noodles.

Pork Tenderloin with Mustard and Rosemary: Rub a pork tenderloin with Dijon mustard, fresh rosemary, salt, and pepper. Roast in the oven until fully cooked, and serve with a side of roasted potatoes and carrots.

SOUPS SALADS AND SIDE DISH

Tomato Basil Soup: Saute canned diced tomatoes in garlic-infused oil, then blend with chicken broth, fresh basil, salt, and pepper. Serve hot with a side of gluten-free croutons.

Mixed Greens Salad: Combine mixed greens with sliced cucumbers, cherry tomatoes, shredded carrots, and a low FODMAP salad dressing (e.g., olive oil and balsamic vinegar).

Roasted Root Vegetables: Toss diced carrots, parsnips, and potatoes with garlic-infused oil, salt, and pepper. Roast in the oven until tender and caramelized.

Quinoa Salad with Cucumber and Mint: Cook quinoa in chicken broth, then toss with diced cucumbers, chopped mint, olive oil, and lemon juice.

Steamed Green Beans with Almonds: Steam fresh green beans until tender, then toss with toasted slivered almonds, olive oil, salt, and pepper.

Butternut Squash Soup: Roast diced butternut squash with olive oil, salt, and pepper, then blend with chicken broth, ginger, and a splash of coconut milk. Serve hot with a side of gluten-free bread.

Greek Salad: Combine romaine lettuce, cherry tomatoes, sliced cucumbers, kalamata olives, feta cheese, and a low FODMAP salad dressing (e.g., olive oil and red wine vinegar).

Remember to always check the ingredients of any pre-made dressings, sauces or condiments you use to make sure they are low FODMAP.

SAUCES

There are many low FODMAP sauces available, or you can make your own using low FODMAP ingredients. Here are some options:

Tomato Sauce: Look for a tomato sauce without added garlic or onion. Alternatively, you can make your own using canned tomatoes, a little olive oil, and some dried herbs like oregano or basil.

Soy Sauce: Use a gluten-free soy sauce or tamari, which are both low in FODMAP.

Mustard: Choose a plain yellow mustard or a Dijon mustard made with low FODMAP ingredients.

BBQ Sauce: Look for a BBQ sauce without onion or garlic. You can also make your own using low-FODMAP ingredients like tomato paste, brown sugar, vinegar, and Worcestershire sauce.

Mayonnaise: Choose a mayonnaise made with low FODMAP ingredients like egg yolks, vinegar, and oil.

Hot Sauce: Look for a hot sauce without added garlic or onion. Many hot sauces are low FODMAP, but be sure to check the ingredients list.

Pesto: Make your pesto using low-FODMAP ingredients like basil, pine nuts, Parmesan cheese, and olive oil.

Remember to always check the ingredients list and serving sizes before consuming any sauces to ensure they are low FODMAP and suitable for your dietary needs.

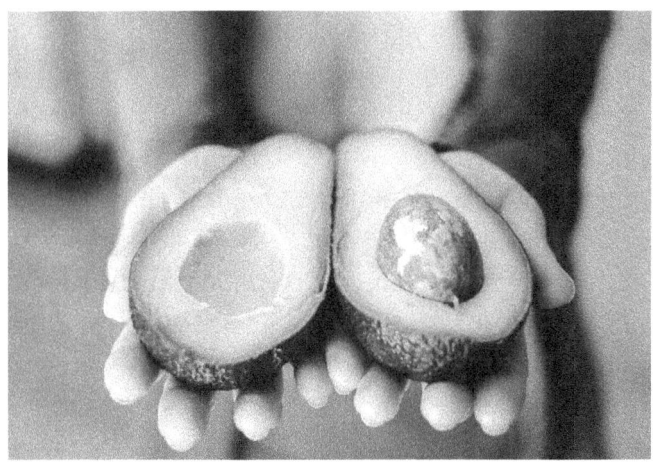

CONCLUSION

In conclusion, the low FODMAP diet is an effective solution for seniors who suffer from digestive issues, such as irritable bowel syndrome (IBS). By eliminating certain types of carbohydrates that are known to trigger symptoms, seniors can experience relief from their digestive issues and improve their overall quality of life.

Cooking and eating on a low FODMAP diet can seem daunting at first, but with the help of this cookbook, seniors can learn to prepare delicious, healthy meals that won't cause discomfort. The recipes in this cookbook are designed to be easy to follow and use simple, readily available ingredients. They also take into account the unique dietary needs of seniors, such as lower sodium and easy-to-chew options.

The cookbook covers a range of dishes, from breakfast to dinner, and includes snacks and desserts as well. Seniors can enjoy favorites like pancakes, lasagna, and muffins without worrying about their digestive symptoms. Additionally, the cookbook includes tips and suggestions for modifying recipes to suit individual needs and preferences.

In addition to providing delicious recipes, this cookbook also offers valuable information about the low FODMAP diet and how it works. Seniors can learn about the different types of FODMAPs and which foods to avoid, as well as how to properly reintroduce these foods after the elimination phase. The cookbook also emphasizes the importance of working with a healthcare professional or registered dietitian to ensure the diet is being implemented correctly and safely.

Implementing a low FODMAP diet can have numerous benefits for seniors beyond just alleviating digestive issues. By reducing symptoms like bloating, gas, and abdominal pain, seniors can experience better sleep, increased energy, and improved mental clarity. Additionally, by choosing whole, nutrient-dense foods as part of the low FODMAP diet, seniors can improve their overall nutrition and potentially reduce the risk of chronic diseases such as heart disease and diabetes.

It's important to note that the low FODMAP diet is not a long-term solution, but rather a temporary elimination and reintroduction of certain foods. Seniors should work with their healthcare professional or registered dietitian to determine the appropriate length of time for the elimination phase and when to start reintroducing FODMAPs back into their diet.

Overall, this low FODMAP cookbook for seniors provides a practical and delicious approach to improving digestive health. By utilizing the recipes and tips in this cookbook, seniors can enjoy a wide variety of flavorful meals without sacrificing their comfort or nutritional needs. Additionally, the cookbook empowers seniors with knowledge and understanding of the low FODMAP diet, which can lead to long-term improvements in their digestive health and overall well-being.

www.ingramcontent.com/pod-product-compliance
Lightning Source LLC
Chambersburg PA
CBHW072236230526
45466CB00024B/2073